SUPPLEMENT FOR PCOS WOMEN

BRAGG HEALTHY LIFESTYLE BOOK

GODBLESS BAKPA AMREVWODJE

Details in this book.

You undertake to indemnify the Author from and against all damages, costs, and expenses, including any legal fees, that may arise from the use of any of the information contained in this book by using its contents and information. You acknowledge that the author disclaims all responsibility for any loss, harm, or damage you may experience. This disclaimer is applicable to any loss, damage, or injury resulting from the use or application of any advice or information provided, whether directly or indirectly, and regardless of whether it results from the breach of a contract, tort, negligence, personal injury, criminal intent, or under any other legal theory.

Other cause of action:

You acknowledge that using the information in this book involves some risk.

By continuing to read this book, you acknowledge that before using any of the recommended treatments, techniques, or information in this book, you should, as appropriate and/or necessary, seek professional advice (including but not limited to your doctor, attorney, financial advisor, or such other advisor as needed).

Table of Contents

INTRODUCTION

Polycystic ovarian syndrome, a common hormonal disease affecting women of reproductive age, menstrual irregularities, excessive hair growth, acne, and obesity are among signs. Infertility, type 2 diabetes, and heart disease are further problems of PCOS. Medications, hormonal therapies, and lifestyle modifications are frequently used as treatments.

Women thirteen years of age and older are susceptible to PCOS. Both the mother and father carry the PCOS-causing gene, and the condition is genetically transmitted from parents to children. Basically, even though it is impossible for your father to get PCOS himself, if he carries the gene, he may have passed it on to you.

In addition, if your mother has PCOS, or if her mother or grandmother did, she might have passed it on to you. However, this does not indicate that the gene vanishes. The sickness might also skip generations. In the following generation, the gene may become active again after going dormant in the current generation.

Hormone balance is thrown off in women who have PCOS. An estrogen level that is too low might occasionally be found in PCOS patients. Overproduction of the male hormone does occur occasionally (androgen).

Androgen and estrogen are chemicals found in the bodies of both men and women. To live regularly, a person has to have a healthy balance between the two types of hormones.

The occurrence of signs like balding or acne may be unexpected if the body's normal hormonal balance is upset.

Patients with PCOS should focus on altering their lifestyle, eating habits, and level of activity. Similar to rheumatism, PCOS actually has no empirical solution and, if not properly managed, might cause discomfort in your life. You can lessen the effects of PCOS by adhering to these basic dietary recommendations along with receiving the appropriate therapy and seeing your doctor on a regular basis.

1. 90% of the time, go for whole foods instead of processed foods. We are aware that many people consume less whole foods because preparing food at home takes time and often requires expensive natural ingredients.

However, it should be highlighted that the more whole foods you consume, the better you will feel, and over time, this will undoubtedly assist lower the costs of treating your disease with medication.

And don't you think your body merits more than just the typical fast food takeout? Even if eating processed food and fast food makes you sicker, you will still end up spending more money because you will regularly visit a hospital or your doctor's office.

2. The total number of calories you consume each day is crucial. You should be conscious of how many calories, fat, protein, and carbohydrates you are putting into your body each day. The greatest foods for weight loss or weight maintenance can be found using meal charts and calorie counting resources.

3. Spend more money on organic foods from nearby farmers. Organic foods may be more expensive, but you will benefit greatly from the fact that they are not laced with antibiotics, pesticides, and other harmful chemicals that can further disrupt your hormone levels. Yes, food-related compounds do have that ability.

CHAPTER 1

CAUSES OF PCOS

Although the precise origin of polycystic ovarian syndrome (PCOS) is uncertain, it is believed to be connected to aberrant hormone levels.

SENSITIVITY TO INSULIN

The hormone insulin is produced by the pancreas to control blood sugar levels. It facilitates the movement of blood glucose into cells, where it is metabolized to provide energy.

Insulin resistance is the term used to describe tissues' resistance to insulin's effects. As a result, the body must generate more insulin to make up for the loss.

The ovaries overproduce testosterone in response to high insulin levels, which interferes with the growth of follicles—the sacs in the ovaries where eggs develop—and hinders proper ovulation.

Weight gain brought on by insulin resistance can exacerbate the symptoms of PCOS because excess fat stimulates the body to create more insulin.

HORMONE DYSREGULATION

It is discovered that many women with PCOS have a hormonal imbalance, particularly in:

1. Increased levels of testosterone, a hormone that is typically produced in modest amounts by all women but is frequently thought of as a male hormone.

2. High levels of luteinizing hormone (LH) – this promotes ovulation but, if levels are too high, may have an inappropriate effect on the ovaries

3. Low levels of sex hormone-binding globulin (SHBG) – a protein in the blood that binds to testosterone and lessens its effect

4. Elevated levels of prolactin, a hormone that increases the production of milk by the breast glands during pregnancy (only in certain women with PCOS).

It is unknown why these hormonal alterations take place specifically.

According to some theories, the issue may have its roots in the ovary, other glands that make these hormones, or the area of the brain that regulates their synthesis.

The alterations might also be brought on by insulin resistance.

Genetics

PCOS can run in families due to genetics. If your mother, sister, or aunt has PCOS, you often have a higher probability of developing it yourself.

This suggests that the condition may have a hereditary component, even though specific genes linked to PCOS have not yet been identified.

CHAPTER 2

COMMON SYMPTOMS OF PCOS

There are many typical PCOS symptoms and indicators in females. This is due to the complexity of PCOS, also known as polycystic ovary syndrome, an endocrine disorder. Basically, it is brought on by abnormal testosterone secretion, which is typical of men. As a result, women exhibit numerous traits that are typically associated with men. Having hair grow in odd areas like the back, face, chest, or tummy is undoubtedly upsetting. Many PCOS patients also experience depression.

Unfortunately, there are other symptoms that are just as upsetting. Hair loss similar to male pattern baldness, obesity, snoring, ovarian cysts, acne, high blood pressure, and localized thickening of the skin are possible. The minor ones are these. Even more sad is infertility brought on by erratic menstrual cycles.

Polycystic ovary syndrome is how common? Researchers estimate that 5% to 10% of women who are able to have children suffer from PCOS. Not everyone will exhibit the same symptoms, and some people will only show minor symptoms while others will show more severe ones. However, everyone often experiences bodily changes and health issues, such as an inability to correctly digest blood sugar, which can result in diabetes and heart disorders. Although there are drugs out there, they simply mitigate PCOS's symptoms. There is currently no known treatment for the illness.

Race and nationality are not factors in PCOS. Because some of the reported victims have relatives who also have the disorder, researchers believe that hereditary factors may be involved. Genetics, however, hasn't been shown in any concrete ways as yet.

Although an imbalance in the secretion of androgens is medically proved to be the cause of the physical changes and health issues experienced by women with PCOS, the exact source of the condition is still unknown. Adolescence is typically when symptoms first arise, and they persist until adulthood.

Since PCOS is a hormonal issue, its consequences are extensive and put sufferers at risk for a wide range of associated ailments. Women with PCOS who do not have normal menstrual cycles are more likely to develop endometrial cancer. Most likely, doctors will advise taking drugs to control menstrual cycles. A proper diet and consistent exercise will be very beneficial for the other known consequences, such as diabetes, high cholesterol, obesity, metabolic syndrome, heart disease, and the like.

Finding a professional with whom a woman can feel at ease and who can offer suitable advice and treatment is crucial for those who have been diagnosed with PCOS. Most importantly, individuals need to educate themselves on the typical PCOS symptoms because doing so will enable them to better combat the illness's crippling effects.

GETTING PREGNANT WITH PCOS

PCOS, also known as polycystic ovarian syndrome, is a relatively prevalent illness that affects up to 10% of females between the ages of 12 and 46. Infertility is brought on by this disorder, which prevents ovulation. However, as PCOS is a curable disorder, it is extremely likely that a woman with the syndrome can conceive. Despite the prevalence of the disorder, no single reason has been identified; instead, researchers think a mix of elements including an excess of insulin, genetics, and inflammation may be to blame.

Treatment for PCOS focuses on controlling the condition so that you can control your ovulation and become pregnant. Changes in lifestyle, such as healthy diet, exercise, and weight loss, are one method of treating the illness (if overweight). Reducing sugar intake and excess weight naturally lowers testosterone and insulin levels, restoring a woman's ovulation and increasing the likelihood of conception. Your doctor may also recommend Metformin, a medication that is frequently prescribed to people with type 2 diabetes to lower insulin levels and encourage ovulation. Additionally, one should modify one's lifestyle. Normally, Metformin is administered for about six months, which is the approximate length of time it may take to start experiencing regular ovulation.

Before attempting to become pregnant with PCOS, it is essential to work closely with your doctor to confirm that you are consistently ovulating because women with PCOS have a greater chance of miscarriages. Therefore, learning how to use a basal thermometer to track your ovulation is essential if you want to know when and whether you ovulate every month. Your doctor will advise that you and your partner try for a baby once the diet and medication have made your ovulation regular.

It is helpful if you and your spouse consult with your doctor frequently to ensure that you can successfully conceive while dealing with PCOS. Despite having PCOS, several women have had healthy children; however, they diligently collaborated with healthcare providers to ensure that their condition was under control before trying to conceive. Your chances of getting pregnant and carrying the baby to term is very high once your doctor has you ovulating regularly for several months.

Diet, maintaining a healthy weight, and exercise are three important aspects of managing PCOS. Even with all three used together, PCOS patients may still require medication in order to become pregnant. This is because your hormones must be in balance for your body to ovulate regularly. One advantage of PCOS that many women have discovered is that it helps their menstrual cycles become more regular if they have given birth safely and maintain a healthy weight and diet. As a result, after their PCOS is under control, many couples go on to have more children.

CHAPTER 3

PCOS DIETARY SUPPLEMENTS

A. Inositol: Inositol is a carbohydrate that is similar to glucose and is found in many foods. Studies have shown that inositol can help regulate ovulation and improve insulin sensitivity in women with PCOS.

B. N-Acetyl Cysteine (NAC): NAC is an antioxidant that can help reduce inflammation and improve ovulation in women with PCOS. It may also help to reduce symptoms of depression and anxiety associated with PCOS.

C. Vitamin D: Vitamin D is important for overall health and has been shown to improve insulin sensitivity and reduce symptoms of depression in women with PCOS.

D. Omega-3 Fatty Acids: Omega-3 fatty acids can help to reduce inflammation and improve insulin sensitivity in women with PCOS. They may also help to reduce symptoms of depression and anxiety associated with PCOS.

E. Chromium: Chromium is a mineral that can help to improve insulin sensitivity and reduce symptoms of depression in women with PCOS.

F. Vitex (Chasteberry): Vitex is an herb that can help to regulate menstrual cycles and reduce symptoms of depression and anxiety associated with PCOS.

It's important to note that supplements are not a replacement for medical treatment, and it's best to consult with a healthcare professional before starting any supplement regimen.

It's important to note that not all supplements may be effective for all women with PCOS, and it's important to consult with a healthcare professional before starting any supplement regimen. It is also important to note that some supplements may interact with other medications you are taking, so it is important to inform your healthcare professional of any supplements you are taking. Supplements should also be taken at the recommended dosages and under the guidance of a healthcare professional.

It's also important to note that while supplements may help manage symptoms of PCOS, they are not a replacement for other treatments such as lifestyle changes, medications and other therapies. For example, Inositol may help with insulin sensitivity, but if a woman's insulin resistance is severe, medication may be necessary to address it. Similarly, Vitex may help regulate menstrual cycles but if cycles are very irregular, other treatments may be necessary to regulate them.

Finally, it is important to remember that while supplements may be able to help manage symptoms of PCOS, they are not a cure for the condition. With the help of a healthcare professional, it is possible to manage PCOS and improve overall health. It's important to continue monitoring symptoms and consulting with a healthcare professional to ensure that the chosen treatment plan is effective.

BENEFITS OF PCOS SUPPLEMENTS

The symptoms of PCOS can be effectively managed with the aid of PCOS supplements. The main advantages of PCOS supplements are that they can assist in regulating hormones, reducing inflammation, and providing vital nutrients that are frequently deficient in PCOS sufferers.

1. Balance Hormones: One of the main goals of PCOS supplements is to assist in hormone balancing, which is essential for treating PCOS symptoms. They might include substances like Vitex, Chasteberry, and Saw Palmetto, which have been demonstrated to lower androgens and assist in controlling estrogen levels.

2. Reduce Inflammation: A typical symptom of PCOS, inflammation can be reduced with the aid of PCOS supplements. Fish oil, omega-3 fatty acids, and curcumin are examples of ingredients with anti-inflammatory effects that can help reduce inflammation and enhance general health.

3. Reduce Insulin Resistance: A frequent symptom of PCOS, insulin resistance, can be reduced with the aid of PCOS supplements. It has been demonstrated that components including inositol, chromium, and magnesium can enhance insulin sensitivity and help control blood sugar levels.

4. Provide Essential Nutrients: PCOS pills offer vital nutrients that a woman's diet can be deficient in. These critical nutrients, which are crucial for overall health and wellbeing, include vitamins, minerals, and antioxidants.

5. Enhances Fertility: Supplements for PCOS can also aid in enhancing fertility. It has been demonstrated that components like zinc, selenium, and folic acid increase ovulation and egg quality, which can aid people with PCOS in getting pregnant.

6. Mood Control: PCOS supplements can also assist with mood control. It has been demonstrated that ingredients like 5-HTP (5-hydroxytryptophan), l-theanine, and ashwagandha can promote sleep, lower anxiety, and uplift mood in general.

7. Improve Skin Health: Supplements for PCOS can also aid in skin health improvement. Zinc, vitamin A, and vitamin E are among the ingredients that can help clear up acne and even out skin tone.

8. Increase Energy Levels: Supplements for PCOS can also assist to increase energy levels. Coenzyme Q10 (CoQ10), B vitamins, and ashwagandha, among other ingredients, have been demonstrated to lessen fatigue, enhance mental clarity, and boost general energy levels.

9. Decrease Bloating: PCOS supplements can also aid in deflating and reducing fluid retention. Horsetail and dandelion root are examples of ingredients that can aid in digestion improvement and bloating reduction.

10. Stop Hair Loss: Supplements for PCOS can also stop hair loss. Saw palmetto, biotin, and zinc are among the ingredients that can help stop hair loss and promote hair growth.

DOSAGE AND SAFETY

A. Recommended dosages for supplements: The recommended dosages for supplements can vary depending on the supplement and the individual. It's important to consult with a healthcare professional for guidance on the appropriate dosage.

B. Potential side effects: While supplements for PCOS are generally considered safe, they can cause side effects in some individuals. These can include stomach upset, headaches, or allergic reactions. If you experience any side effects, it's important to stop taking the supplement and consult with a healthcare professional.

C. Interactions with other medications: Some supplements for PCOS may interact with other medications you are taking. It's important to inform your healthcare professional of any supplements you are taking and to check for potential interactions with any other medications.

It's important to note that the safety and effectiveness of supplements may not be fully understood and more research is needed. Also, supplements are not regulated by the FDA as medications are, so it's important to buy supplements from reputable sources and to be cautious when taking them.

Additionally, it's important to note that some supplements may not be suitable for certain individuals such as pregnant or breastfeeding women, or those with certain medical conditions. It's important to consult with a healthcare professional before starting any supplement regimen, especially if you have any pre-existing medical conditions.

It's also important to remember that just because a supplement is natural or "organic" does not mean it is automatically safe. Some natural supplements can have serious side effects and interactions with other medications. Therefore, it is important to consult with a healthcare professional before taking any natural supplements.

Finally, it is worth mentioning that some supplements may be counterfeit or adulterated, so it's important to buy supplements from reputable sources. Some of the reputable sources are from reputable pharmacies, health food stores, or online retailers. It is also important to check the label for the supplement's ingredients and the dosage per pill.

CHAPTER 4

LIFESTYLE CHANGES FOR PCOS

A. DIET AND NUTRITION:

Low Glycemic Index (GI) diet: A low-GI diet can help to regulate blood sugar levels, which can be beneficial for women with PCOS. This diet includes eating foods with a low glycemic index such as whole grains, fruits, vegetables, and lean protein.

High Fiber diet: Eating a high-fiber diet can help to regulate blood sugar levels and promote weight loss, which can be beneficial for women with PCOS. Foods high in fiber include fruits, vegetables, whole grains, and legumes. Adequate Protein intake: Adequate protein intake is important for maintaining muscle mass and promoting weight loss, which can be beneficial for women with PCOS.

B. EXERCISE:

Importance of regular exercise: Regular exercise is important for overall health and can help to regulate blood sugar levels, promote weight loss, and reduce symptoms of depression and anxiety associated with PCOS.

Types of exercises recommended for PCOS: Aerobic exercises such as brisk walking, cycling, and swimming, and resistance training such as weightlifting, and yoga are recommended for women with PCOS.

C. STRESS MANAGEMENT:

Importance of managing stress: Stress can worsen symptoms of PCOS and increase the risk of developing certain health conditions such as diabetes and heart disease.

Techniques for managing stress: Techniques for managing stress include exercise, meditation, mindfulness, and yoga, as well as talking to a therapist or counselor.

It's important to note that while these lifestyle changes can be beneficial in managing symptoms of PCOS, they should be combined with other treatments such as medications and supplements under the guidance of a healthcare professional.

Additionally, it's important to remember that making lifestyle changes can be challenging, especially when it comes to diet and exercise. It's important to set realistic goals and take small steps towards making changes. Consulting a dietitian or fitness professional can help create a personalized plan that fits your needs and lifestyle.

It's also important to note that stress management is a crucial aspect of managing PCOS, as stress can exacerbate symptoms and contribute to the development of certain health conditions. Finding healthy ways to manage stress, such as yoga, meditation, and therapy, is important for overall well-being.

The fact that everyone is unique means that what works for one person might not necessarily work for another. It's important to be patient and persistent with lifestyle changes and to consult with a healthcare professional for guidance and support.

Finally, it's important to remember that these lifestyle changes should be part of an overall treatment plan for PCOS, which may also include medications and supplements under the guidance of a healthcare professional. With the help of a healthcare professional, it is possible to manage PCOS and improve overall health.

CHAPTER 5

ADDITIONAL THERAPIES

A. HERBAL REMEDIES

Saw Palmetto: Saw Palmetto is an herb that may help to reduce symptoms of hirsutism (excessive hair growth) and acne associated with PCOS.

Green Tea: Green tea contains antioxidants and has anti-inflammatory properties that may help to improve insulin sensitivity and reduce symptoms of PCOS.

Turmeric: Turmeric is an herb that has anti-inflammatory properties and may help to improve insulin sensitivity and reduce symptoms of PCOS.

B. Acupuncture: Acupuncture is a form of traditional Chinese medicine that involves the insertion of thin needles into specific points on the body. It may help to reduce symptoms of PCOS such as irregular menstrual cycles and infertility.

C. Naturopathy: Naturopathy is a holistic approach to health that focuses on the use of natural remedies, such as herbs and supplements, to promote well-being. Naturopathic practitioners may recommend a combination of therapies such as diet and lifestyle changes, herbal remedies, and supplements to manage symptoms of PCOS.

It's important to note that the effectiveness of these therapies in treating PCOS may not be fully understood, and more research is needed. Also, it's important to consult with a healthcare professional before trying any alternative therapies, as they may interact with other medications or may not be suitable for certain individuals.

It's also important to note that while these therapies may be helpful in managing symptoms of PCOS, they are not a replacement for medical treatment. With the help of a healthcare professional, it is possible to manage PCOS and improve overall health. It's important to continue monitoring symptoms and consulting with a healthcare professional to ensure that the chosen treatment plan is effective.

It's also important to note that herbal remedies and supplements can have side effects and may interact with other medications, so it's important to use them under the guidance of a healthcare professional. It's also important to make sure that you are buying from reputable sources and that the product is of high quality.

It's also worth mentioning that acupuncture and naturopathy may not be covered by insurance, so it's important to check with your insurance provider to see what is covered and what out-of-pocket costs you may incur.

Finally, it's important to remember that these therapies should be part of an overall treatment plan for PCOS, which may also include medications, lifestyle changes and supplements under the guidance of a healthcare professional. With the help of a healthcare professional, it is possible to manage PCOS and improve overall health.

MONITORING PROGRESS:

A. Tracking symptoms: It's important to keep track of symptoms of PCOS such as menstrual cycles, weight changes, and hirsutism, in order to monitor the effectiveness of the treatment plan.

B. Monitoring hormonal levels: Hormonal imbalances are a key feature of PCOS, so it's important to monitor hormonal levels such as testosterone, estrogen, and luteinizing hormone (LH) to ensure that the treatment plan is effective.

C. Assessing fertility: PCOS can affect fertility, so it's important to monitor fertility by tracking ovulation and assessing the effectiveness of any fertility treatments that may be part of the treatment plan.

It's important to work closely with a healthcare professional to monitor progress and make adjustments to the treatment plan as needed. Regular check-ins with a healthcare professional can help ensure that the treatment plan is effective and that any issues or side effects are addressed promptly.

It's also important to remember that PCOS is a chronic condition, and managing symptoms may require ongoing monitoring and adjustments to the treatment plan.

CHAPTER 6

MEAL PLAN FOR PCOS

Day 1:

Breakfast: Chia-seed-infused overnight oats with almond milk and fresh berries.

Snack: Apple slices with almond butter.

Lunch: Kale salad with roasted sweet potatoes, quinoa, avocado, and grilled salmon

Snack: Greek yogurt infused fresh fruit, and nuts.

Dinner: Roasted broccoli and cauliflower and baked cod

Day 2:

Breakfast: scrambled eggs with mushrooms and spinach.

Snack: Hummus-topped celery sticks.

Lunch: Stir-fried shrimp and vegetables over brown rice

Snack: Roasted chickpeas

Dinner: Grilled chicken with roasted asparagus and a sweet potato.

Day 3:

Breakfast: Oatmeal with blueberries and walnuts

Snack: Hard-boiled eggs

Lunch: A wrap of vegetables with hummus, tomatoes, cucumbers, and avocado.

Snack: Unsweetened Greek yogurt with fresh berries

Dinner: Quinoa with salmon and roasted Brussels sprouts.

Day 4:

Breakfast: Chia seeds, banana, and almond butter in a smoothie bowl.

Snack: Sliced peaches and cottage cheese.

Lunch: lentil soup with a side salad

Snack: Celery sticks with peanut butter.

Dinner: Baked salmon with roasted Brussels sprouts and a sweet potato

Day 5:

Breakfast: scrambled eggs and vegetables

Snack: Hummus and carrots

Lunch: Turkey wrap with lettuce, tomato, and avocado

Snack: Chia seeds added to Greek yogurt.

Dinner: Baked cod with roasted broccoli and cauliflower

Day 6:

Breakfast: Overnight oats with almond milk, banana, and walnuts

Snack: Slices of apples with almond butter.

Lunch: quinoa salad with grilled chicken and green vegetables

Snack: roasted chickpeas

Dinner: grilled chicken with roasted asparagus and a sweet potato

Day 7:

Breakfast: Chia seeds, banana, and almond butter in a smoothie bowl.

Snack: cooked eggs

Lunch: A wrap of vegetables with hummus, tomatoes, cucumbers, and avocado.

Snack: Unflavored Greek yogurt and fresh berries.

Dinner: baked salmon with roasted Brussels sprouts and a sweet potato

CHAPTER 7

RECIPES

1. Ginger Pear Overnight Oats:

Ingredients: Half a cup of rolled oats, half a cup of almond milk, diced half a pear, one tablespoon maple syrup, half tablespoon grated ginger, two teaspoons of walnuts, chopped **and** two tablespoons of dried cranberries

Instructions:

1. Combine the oats, almond milk, pear dice, ginger, and maple syrup in a bowl.

2. Put it in the fridge and let it there for the night.

3. Add chopped walnuts and dried cranberries on top in the morning. Enjoy!

Prep. Time: Five minutes

Time to Relax: Eight hours

2. Kale and Feta Egg Muffins:

Ingredients: Six big eggs ,one cup chopped kale, two teaspoons olive oil, One-fourth teaspoon ground black pepper; one-fourth cup feta cheese

Instructions:

1. Turn on the oven to 400°F.

2. Use olive oil to coat a muffin pan.

3. Evenly distribute the chopped kale among the muffin tin's cups.

4. Combine the eggs, feta cheese, and freshly ground black pepper in a bowl.

5. Fill each cup in the muffin tin with two-third of the egg mixture.

6. Bake the eggs for fifteen minutes, or until they are fully set.

7. Enjoy your Kale and Feta Egg Muffins!

Prep Time: Ten minutes

Bake Time: Fifteen minutes

3. Smoothie with chocolate and peanut butter:

Ingredients: One banana, frozen, half cup almond milk, one tablespoon of organic peanut butter, one teaspoon cocoa powder, one teaspoon of honey

Instructions:

1. Blend the frozen banana with the almond milk, peanut butter, honey, and chocolate powder.

2. Blend until completely smooth.

3. Serve and enjoy your Chocolate Peanut Butter Smoothie!

Prep Time: Five minutes

4. Egg on Avocado Toast:

Ingredients: Two slices of whole wheat bread, half a mashed avocado, one-fourth teaspoon dried garlic, One-fourth teaspoon of ground black pepper, two eggs

Instructions:

1. Toast the bread and cover each piece with the mashed avocado.

2. Add some freshly ground black pepper and garlic powder.

3. Put a nonstick skillet on the stovetop at medium heat.

4. Once the whites are set, crack the eggs into the skillet and cook for a few minutes.

5. Top the avocado toast with the eggs and eat.

Prep Time: Five minutes

Cooking Time: Five minutes.

5. Eggs with Sweet Potato Hash:

Ingredients: one diced sweet potato, two tablespoons of olive oil, and one-fourth teaspoon of garlic powder, one-fourth teaspoon of ground black pepper, two eggs

Instructions:

1. Olive oil should be warmed in a nonstick skillet over medium heat.

2. Add the chopped sweet potato and season with freshly ground black pepper and garlic powder.

3. Cook the sweet potatoes for ten to fifteen minutes, or until they are soft.

4. Once the whites are set, crack the eggs into the skillet and cook for a few minutes.

5. Arrange the eggs on top of the sweet potato hash and serve.

Prep Time: Five minutes

Time to Cook: Fifteen minutes

6. Greek Yogurt Parfait:

Ingredients: One cup of greek yogurt, one-fourth cup of granola, one-fourth cup of fresh berries, one teaspoon of honey

Instructions:

1. Combine the Greek yogurt, granola, and fresh fruit in a bowl.

2. Drizzle everything with honey and combine.

3. Dish up your greek yogurt parfait and savor it!

Prep Time: Five minutes

7. Oatmeal with peanut butter and bananas:

Ingredients: One banana, sliced, half cup rolled oats, half cup almond milk, two teaspoons of peanut butter, one teaspoon of honey

Instructions:

1. Bring the almond milk to a boil in a pot.

2. Stir in the rolled oats.

3. Simmer for five minutes while occasionally stirring.

4. Turn off the heat and whisk in the honey, peanut butter, and banana slices.

5. Serve your Peanut Butter and Banana Oatmeal and enjoy!

Prep Time: Five minutes

Cooking Time: Five minutes

8. Spinach and Tomato Omelet:

Ingredients: Two tablespoons olive oil, one cup chopped spinach, half cup halved cherry tomatoes, three big eggs, one-fourth teaspoon black pepper, ground

Instructions:

1 Olive oil should be warmed in a nonstick skillet over medium heat.

2. Include the cherry tomatoes and spinach, and simmer for a few minutes, or until the spinach is wilted.

3. Combine the eggs and freshly ground black pepper in a bowl.

4. When the eggs are ready, pour the egg mixture into the skillet and simmer for a few minutes.

5. Dish up your spinach and tomato omelet and savor it!

Prep Time: Five minutes

Cooking Time: Five minutes

9. Chia Seed Pudding:

Ingredients: One cup almond milk, one tablespoon honey, one-fourth teaspoon crushed cinnamon, half cup chia seeds, one-fourth cup of fresh berries.

Instructions:

1. Combine the chia seeds, almond milk, honey, and cinnamon powder in a bowl.

2. Combine everything and let it set for at least 4 hours or overnight in the refrigerator.

3. Arrange some fresh berries on top of the chia seed pudding and enjoy.

Prep Time: Five minutes

Time to Relax: Four hours

10. Banana and Almond Butter Toast:

Ingredients: One sliced banana and two pieces of whole wheat bread, two teaspoons of almond butter.

Instructions:

1. After toasting the bread, smear each piece with almond butter.

2. Add the banana slices on top.

3. Present and savor your toast with banana and almond butter!

Prep Time: Five minutes

LUNCH

1. Quinoa Veggie Bowl:

Ingredients: Half cup quinoa, half cup cooked chickpeas, one-fourth cup halved cherry tomatoes, one-fourth cup chopped cucumber, one-fourth cup chopped red bell pepper, three tablespoons diced red onion, one teaspoon Dijon mustard, one teaspoon chopped garlic, two tablespoons olive oil, one tablespoon balsamic vinegar, and salt and pepper to taste.

Instructions:

1. As specified on the packaging, prepare the quinoa.

2. Toss together the cooked quinoa, chickpeas, tomatoes, cucumber, bell pepper, and red onion in a large mixing bowl.

3. Whisk together the olive oil, balsamic vinegar, mustard, garlic, salt, and pepper in a small basin.

4. Toss the quinoa mixture with the dressing to blend.

5. You may serve the quinoa veggie bowl hot or chilled.

Prep Time: Fifteen minutes

2. Salmon Baked with Avocado:

Ingredients: One-fourth teaspoon garlic powder, four (four-ounce) salmon fillets, one tablespoon onion powder one tablespoon chili powder paprika, half teaspoon, half teaspoon cumin powder, to taste salt and pepper , two tablespoons olive oil, one peeled and diced avocado

Instructions:

1. Preheat the oven to 400°F (200 degrees C).

2. On a baking pan, place the salmon fillets.

3. Combine the garlic powder, onion powder, chili powder, paprika, and cumin in a small mixing dish. Sprinkle the mixture over the salmon. Season with salt and pepper.

4. Drizzle the salmon with olive oil.

5. Bake for twelve to fifteen minutes or until the salmon is cooked through.

6. Garnish the salmon with diced avocado.

Prep Time: Ten minutes

3. Egg White Omelet with Spinach and Feta:

Ingredients: Three egg whites, one-fourth cup chopped spinach, one-fourth cup crumbled feta cheese, one tablespoon olive oil, add salt and pepper to taste.

Instructions:

1. In a medium mixing bowl, whisk together the egg whites until light and fluffy.

2. In a skillet set over medium heat, warm the olive oil.

3. Pour the egg whites into the skillet and simmer for two minutes, stirring occasionally.

4. Stir in the spinach and feta until the spinach is wilted and the cheese is melted.

5. Season with salt and pepper and saute for another two minutes.

6. Serve the omelet warm.

Prep Time: Ten minutes

4. Mediterranean Quinoa Salad:

Ingredients: One-fourth cup chopped cucumber, one-fourth cup cooked quinoa, one-fourth cup chopped red bell pepper, one-fourth cup pitted and halved kalamata olives, two tablespoons olive oil, two teaspoons fresh lemon, one tablespoon minced fresh parsley, one teaspoon dried oregano, add salt and pepper to taste

Instructions:

1. Toss together the cooked quinoa, tomatoes, cucumber, bell pepper, and olives in a large mixing basin.

2. Whisk together the olive oil, lemon juice, parsley, and oregano in a small basin.

3. Pour the dressing over the quinoa mixture and toss to incorporate.

4. Add pepper and salt to taste.

5. Serve the Mediterranean quinoa salad cold.

Prep Time: Ten minutes

5. Grilled Chicken with Vegetables:

Ingredients: Four boneless, skinless chicken breasts, half red bell pepper sliced, half yellow bell pepper sliced, half onion sliced, one teaspoon minced garlic, one teaspoon chili powder, one teaspoon smoked paprika, one teaspoon cumin powder, two tablespoons olive oil, add salt and pepper to taste.

Instructions:

1. Preheat the grill to medium-high heat.

2. In a large mixing bowl, add the bell peppers, onion, garlic, chili powder, smoked paprika, cumin, and olive oil.

3. Toss to incorporate and season with salt and pepper.

4. Grill the chicken and veggies for eight to ten minutes, turning periodically, or until the chicken is cooked through and the vegetables are soft.

5. Serve the grilled chicken and vegetables warm.

Prep Time: Ten minutes

6. Roasted Veggie Bowl with Hummus:

Ingredients: Half cup broccoli florets, half cup cauliflower florets, half cup cherry tomatoes halved, half cup diced red onion, two tablespoons olive oil, one tablespoon balsamic vinegar, one teaspoon chopped garlic, one-fourth cup hummus, salt and pepper to taste

Instructions:

1. Preheat the oven to 400 degrees F. (200 degrees C).

2. Toss together the broccoli, cauliflower, tomatoes, and red onion in a large mixing basin.

3. Toss the veggies with the olive oil and balsamic vinegar.

4. Arrange the vegetables on a baking sheet and season with garlic, salt, and pepper.

5. Roast for twenty minutes or until the potatoes are soft.

6. Serve the roasted vegetables with hummus.

Prep Time: Ten minutes

7. Zucchini Noodles with Pesto:

Ingredients: Two zucchini, spiralized, two tablespoons olive oil, three tablespoons pesto, one-fourth cup cherry tomatoes halved, one-fourth cup kalamata olives pitted and split, two tablespoons grated parmesan cheese, add salt and pepper to taste.

Instructions:

1. Butter should be melted in a sizable skillet over medium heat.

2. Cook for five minutes, stirring regularly, after adding the zucchini noodles.

3. Stir in the pesto, tomatoes, olives, and Parmesan cheese until mixed.

4. Cook for another two minutes, or until the zucchini noodles are soft.

5. Season with salt and pepper to taste.

6. Serve the zucchini noodles warm.

Prep Time: Ten minutes

8. Greek Salad:

Ingredients: Half head romaine lettuce chopped, one-fourth cup feta cheese crumbled, one-fourth cup cucumber diced, one-fourth cup red onion diced, one-fourth cup pitted and halved kalamata olives ,one-fourth cup halved cherry tomatoes, two tablespoons olive oil, two teaspoons fresh lemon juice, one teaspoon dried oregano, add salt and pepper to taste.

Instructions:

1. Combine the lettuce, feta, cucumber, red onion, olives, and tomatoes in a large mixing basin.

2. Whisk together the olive oil, lemon juice, and oregano in a small basin.

3. Mix the salad after adding the dressing.

4. To taste, add salt and pepper to the food.

5. Serve the Greek salad chilled.

Prep Time: Ten minutes

9. Cauliflower Rice Bowl:

Ingredients: One-fourth cup edamame, one-fourth cup shredded carrots, one-fourth cup chopped red bell pepper, two tablespoons olive oil, one tablespoon tamari, one teaspoon minced garlic, one teaspoon sesame seeds, add salt and pepper to taste.

Instructions:

1. A big skillet with medium heat is used to warm the olive oil.

2. Stir in the cauliflower rice, edamame, carrots, and bell pepper until mixed.

3. Stir in the tamari, garlic, and sesame seeds until mixed.

4. Cook for five minutes, or until the vegetables are soft.

5. Season with salt and pepper to taste.

6. Serve the cauliflower rice bowl warm.

Prep Time: Ten minutes

10 Avocado Toast:

Ingredients: Two slices whole grain bread, one peeled and mashed avocado, one tablespoon olive oil, one teaspoon lemon juice, one-fourth teaspoon garlic powder, one-fourth teaspoon onion powder, one-fourth teaspoon chili powder, add salt and pepper to taste.

Instructions:

1. Toast the bread.

2. Using a fork, mash the avocado in a small bowl.

3. Stir in the olive oil, lemon juice, garlic powder, onion powder, and chili powder. Stir until well blended.

4. Toast is covered in mashed avocado.

5. Season with salt and pepper to taste.

6. Serve the avocado toast warm.

Prep Time: Ten minutes

DINNER

1. Baked salmon with roasted asparagus:

Ingredients: Four (four-ounce) fillets of salmon, one bunch trimmed asparagus; two tablespoons split olive oil; two tablespoons freshly squeezed lemon juice, one teaspoon minced garlic, pepper and salt as desired.

Instructions:

1. Set the oven to 425 degrees.

2. Arrange salmon fillets on a parchment-lined baking pan. Add a drizzle of lemon juice and one tablespoon of olive oil. Add garlic, salt, and pepper.

3. Set out a baking sheet with parchment paper and add the asparagus to it. Sprinkle with pepper and salt after adding the remaining olive oil.

4. Bake the salmon and asparagus on both baking pans for fifteen to twenty minutes, depending on their sizes, to ensure complete cooking.

Pre-Time: Fifteen to twenty minutes

2. Chicken with vegetables in a slow cooker:

Ingredients: Four skinless, boneless chicken breasts, two cups of cubed potatoes; one cup of chopped carrots, one cup of chopped celery, one teaspoon of minced garlic, one cup of low-sodium chicken broth, one teaspoon oregano, add salt and pepper to taste.

Instructions:

1. Fill a slow cooker with chicken breasts.

2. Include potatoes, carrots, celery, onion, garlic, chicken stock, oregano, salt, and pepper. To blend, stir.

3. Cook the chicken and veggies until the chicken is well cooked, about six-seven hours on low or three–four hours on high.

Pre-Time: Six-seven hours (low) or three–four hours (high)

3. Grilled Portobello Mushrooms:

Ingredients: Four large Portobello mushrooms, stems and gills removed, two tablespoons each of olive oil and balsamic vinegar, one teaspoon of minced garlic, and four. Pepper and salt as desired.

Instructions:

1. Increase the heat on the grill to medium-high.

2. Combine olive oil, balsamic vinegar, garlic, salt, and pepper in a small bowl.

3. Use the oil-vinegar mixture to brush on the Portobello mushrooms.

4. Grill the mushrooms for six to eight minutes on each side, or until they are fork-tender.

Six to eight minutes in advance

4. Salad with black beans and quinoa:

Ingredients: One cup cooked quinoa, one can rinsed and drained black beans, one diced red bell pepper, one diced avocado, half cup cherry tomatoes, one teaspoon cumin, two tablespoons olive oil, two tablespoons freshly squeezed lime juice, and salt and pepper to taste

Instructions:

1. Combine the quinoa, black beans, red bell pepper, avocado, and cherry tomatoes in a big bowl.

2. Combine the olive oil, cumin, lime juice, salt, and pepper in a small bowl.

3. Drizzle the quinoa and black bean salad with the oil and lime juice combination, and whisk to incorporate.

Pre-time: Ten minutes

5. Zucchini Noodles with Pesto:

Ingredients: Two tablespoons olive oil, two minced garlic cloves, four medium zucchini, spiralized, one-fourth cup basil pesto, and salt and pepper to taste.

Instructions:

1. In a big skillet over medium-high heat, warm the olive oil.

2. Include the garlic and cook for one minute.

3. Add the noodles, and cook for an additional three to four minutes or until the noodles are soft.

4. Add the pesto and blend.

5. To taste, add salt and pepper to the food.

Pre-Time: five minutes

6. Baked Sweet Potato Fries:

Ingredients: Four strips of sweet potatoes, peeled, two tablespoons of olive oil and one teaspoon of garlic powder. One teaspoon paprika, Salt and pepper to taste

Instructions:

1. Set the oven to 425 degrees.

2. Add olive oil to a big bowl with the sweet potato slices. Coat by tossing.

3. Include paprika, salt, pepper, and garlic powder. Combine by tossing.

4. Arrange the strips of sweet potatoes on a baking sheet covered with parchment paper.

5. Bake sweet potatoes for twenty to twenty five minutes, or until they are crisp and tender.

Twenty to twenty five minutes prior to start

7. Baked Eggplant Parmesan:

Ingredients: Salt and pepper to taste, two big eggplants cut into one fourth-inch rounds, two cups low-sodium marinara sauce, two cups part-skim mozzarella, one-fourth cup freshly grated Parmesan cheese, two tablespoons olive oil, and one teaspoon Italian seasoning

Instructions:

1. Set the oven to 400 degrees.

2. Arrange the slices of eggplant on a baking sheet covered with parchment paper. Add a drizzle of olive oil and season with salt, pepper, and Italian seasoning.

3. Bake the eggplant for fifteen to twenty minutes, or until it is soft.

4. Fill a nine x thirteen (9 * 13) baking dish with half cup of marinara sauce.

5. Spread the marinara sauce on top of half of the eggplant slices. Add one-fourth cup Parmesan cheese and one cup mozzarella cheese on top.

6. Cover the cheese with the remaining slices of eggplant and the remaining marinara sauce the remainder of the mozzarella and parmesan cheese on top.

7. Bake for twenty to twenty five minutes, or until bubbling and melted cheese.

Thirty-five to forty-five minutes prior to start

8. Tacos with Roasted Chickpeas:

Ingredients: Chickpeas cooked in two cups with two tablespoons olive oil, two teaspoons of chili powder, one teaspoon of cumin, and half a teaspoon of garlic powder, eight small corn tortillas, salt and pepper to taste, sliced tomatoes, avocado, cilantro, and shredded lettuce for garnish

Instructions:

1. Set the oven to 400 degrees.

2. Spread the chickpeas out on a parchment-lined baking sheet. Add a drizzle of olive oil and season with salt, pepper, cumin, chili powder, and garlic powder.

3. Bake the chickpeas for twenty to twenty five minutes, or until they are crispy.

4. In the meantime, warm the tortillas over a medium heat in a skillet.

5. Fill warmed tortillas with roasted chickpeas and top with chosen garnishes to construct tacos.

Twenty five to thirty five minutes prior to start

9. Lentil Soup:

Ingredients: Two tablespoons of olive oil, one diced onion, two minced garlic cloves, two diced carrots, two diced celery stalks, one teaspoon of Italian spice, and two cups of rinsed dried lentils make up this recipe. Low-sodium vegetable broth in six cups, with salt and pepper to taste

Instructions:

1. In a big pot set over medium heat, warm the olive oil.

2. Add the vegetables and simmer for a further five-seven minutes, or until they are cooked.

3. Stir the lentils and Italian seasoning together.

4. Pour the veggie broth into the soup and bring it to a boil. Simmer for twenty to thirty minutes, or until lentils are cooked, on low heat.

5. To taste, add salt and pepper to the food.

Twenty five to thirty five minutes prior to start

10. Quinoa Pilaf with Roasted Veggies:

Ingredients: Three cups of cooked quinoa, one red bell pepper, one red onion, two carrots, one head of broccoli, two tablespoons of olive oil, two tablespoons of freshly squeezed lemon juice, and one-half teaspoon of garlic powder. To taste, add salt and pepper.

Instructions:

1. Set the oven to 400 degrees.

2. Arrange carrots, broccoli, red bell pepper, red onion, and a baking sheet covered with parchment paper. Add some olive oil and season with salt, pepper, and garlic powder.

3. Bake the vegetables for twenty to twenty five minutes, or until they are soft.

4. Combine cooked quinoa, roasted vegetables, lemon juice, salt, and pepper in a large bowl. To blend, stir.

Pre-time: Twenty to thirty minutes

SNACKS:

1. Bark made of dark chocolate and almonds:

Ingredients: One cup chips of dark chocolate, One-fourth cup toasted almonds, two teaspoons each of flaxseed and pumpkin seeds, sunflower seeds, two tablespoons chopped dried apricots, two tablespoons coconut oil.

Instructions:

1. Microwave the chocolate chips and coconut oil for thirty seconds in a microwave-safe bowl.

2. Stir the chocolate and oil until they are melted and blended.

3. Include the almonds, flaxseed, pumpkin, sunflower, and dried apricots. Stir everything together until it is all thoroughly covered in the melted chocolate.

4. Spoon the mixture equally onto a baking sheet that has been lined with parchment paper.

5. Refrigerate the baking sheet for thirty minutes, or until the chocolate is firm.

6. Break the bark into pieces and enjoy once the chocolate has hardened.

Prep Time: Ten minutes

Time to Chill: Thirty minutes

Time total: Forty minutes

2. Roasted Chickpeas:

Ingredients: One (fifteen-ounce) can of washed and drained chickpeas, two tablespoons of olive oil and a teaspoon of garlic powder, one teaspoon each of cumin and smoked paprika, half teaspoon salt, sea.

Instructions:

1. Set the oven to 375 degrees.

2. Use parchment paper to cover a baking sheet.

3. Spread some olive oil over the chickpeas before placing them on the baking pan.

4. Season with sea salt, cumin, smoky paprika, and garlic powder.

5. Combine by tossing.

6. Roast the chickpeas until they are golden brown and crispy for twenty to twenty minutes, tossing once halfway through.

7. Take pleasure in warm or room temperature.

Time to Prepare: Five minutes

Time to Cook: Twenty-twenty five minutes

Total Time: Twenty five-thirty minutes

3. Trail Mix Bites:

Ingredients: One cup of rolled oats and half cup of unsweetened coconut shreds, half cup of almond meal, one fourth cup sunflower seeds, one fourth cup of pumpkin seeds, one fourth cup chopped walnuts, two tablespoons worth of chia seeds, one teaspoon of cinnamon, ground, one-fourth teaspoon sea salt, four cups of honey, and four cups of peanut butter

Instructions:

1. Line a baking sheet with parchment paper and preheat the oven to 350 degrees Fahrenheit.

2. Combine the oats, coconut, almond meal, sunflower, pumpkin, walnut, chia, cinnamon, and salt in a sizable bowl.

3. In another bowl, thoroughly combine the honey and peanut butter.

4. Combine the honey mixture with the oat mixture and whisk to thoroughly combine.

5. Scoop the mixture into one-inch balls and set them on the baking sheet that has been prepared.

6. Bake the bites for twelve to fifteen minutes, or until golden brown.

Let the food cool before serving.

Prep Time: Ten minute

Cooking Time: Twelve–Fifteen minutes

Time: Twenty two to twenty five minutes

4. Toast with sweet potatoes and hummus:

Ingredients: One sweet potato, cut into rounds one and half inches wide, two tablespoons olive oil, sea salt, to taste, two slices gluten-free bread, one-fourth cup hummus

Instructions:

1. Set the oven to 375 degrees.

2. Place the sweet potato slices on a baking sheet and drizzle with olive oil and a pinch of sea salt.

3. Bake for twenty minutes or until the sweet potatoes are soft and golden brown.

4. Toast the bread.

5. Spread the hummus on the toast and top with the roasted sweet potatoes.

6. Enjoy!

Prep Time: Five minutes

Cooking Time: Twenty minutes

Time total: Twenty five minutes

5. Poached Egg on Avocado Toast:

Ingredients: One pitted and chopped avocado, plus one teaspoon of lemon juice, two pieces of gluten-free bread, one teaspoon olive oil, two eggs, and sea salt to taste, two tablespoons white vinegar.

Instructions:

1. Mash the avocado with the lemon juice and a dash of sea salt in a small bowl.

2. The bread is toast.

3. Cover the toast with the mashed avocado.

4. In a little skillet over medium heat, warm the olive oil.

5. Lower the heat to low and crack the eggs into the skillet.

6. After adding the vinegar, cook the eggs for three to four minutes, or until the whites are set.

7. Top the avocado toast with the poached eggs and eat.

Prep Time: Five minutes

Cooking Time: Ten minutes

Total Time: Fifteen minutes

6. Fried zucchini:

Ingredients: Grated two medium zucchini, three tablespoons of almond flour, one tablespoon of chia seeds, one teaspoon of cumin, and one teaspoon of garlic powder, half teaspoon sea salt, one lightly beaten egg and two teaspoons of olive oil.

Instructions:

1. Spoon sea salt over the grated zucchini in a colander.

2. After let it sit for ten minutes, squeeze away any extra moisture.

3. Combine the zucchini, almond flour, chia seeds, cumin, garlic powder, and sea salt in a sizable bowl.

4. Include the egg and stir everything up thoroughly.

5. Place a big skillet over medium heat and warm the olive oil.

6. Form two-inch patties out of the zucchini mixture by scooping it into the griddle.

7. Cook for two to three minutes on each side, or until golden.

8. Present warm, and savor.

Prep Time: Ten minutes

Total Time: Eighteen minutes

7. Bites of apple and almond butter:

Ingredients: Two cored and thinly cut apples, two teaspoons of hemp seeds , one-fourth cup of almond butter, two tablespoons worth of chia seeds

Instructions:

1. Cover each apple slice with the almond butter.

2. Add hemp and chia seeds as garnish.

3. Enjoy!

Prep Time: Five minutes

 Total Time: Five minutes

8. Chocolate-Covered Strawberries:

Ingredients: One pint dried and cleaned strawberries, one cup dark chocolate chips, two tablespoons coconut oil.

Instructions:

1. Use parchment paper to cover a baking sheet.

2. Microwave the chocolate chips and coconut oil for thirty seconds in a bowl that is microwave-safe.

3. Stir the ingredients together until the chocolate and oil are melted.

4. Lay each strawberry on the lined baking sheet after being covered in the molten chocolate.

5. Refrigerate the baking sheet for thirty minutes, or until the chocolate is firm.

6. Enjoy!

Prep Time: Ten minutes

Cooking Time: Thirty minutes

Total Time: Forty minutes

9. Avocado and Cucumber Salad:

Ingredients: Two thinly sliced cucumbers, one diced avocado, one tablespoon olive oil, and one tablespoon lemon juice, to add sea salt taste.

Instructions:

1. Combine the cucumbers, avocado, olive oil, and lemon juice in a big bowl.

2. Add a pinch of sea salt, to taste.

3. Enjoy!

Prep Time: Five minutes

Total Time: Five minutes

10. Sweet potato chips:

Ingredients: Two finely sliced sweet potatoes, two teaspoons of olive oil, to taste, add sea salt

Instructions:

1. Set the oven to 375 degrees.

2. You should line a baking sheet with parchment paper.

3. Arrange the sweet potato slices on the baking sheet, then sprinkle with a little sea salt and drizzle with olive oil.

4. Bake the sweet potatoes for twenty minutes, or until they are crisp and golden brown.

5. Enjoy!

Prep Time: Ten minutes

Cooking Time: Twenty minutes

Approximately Thirty minutes.

DESERTS

1. Cinnamon Apple Crumble:

Ingredients: Two cups of apple slices, half-cup of almond flour, two tablespoons of cinnamon, two tablespoons coconut oil, two teaspoons maple syrup, one-fourth teaspoon of salt.

Instructions:

1. Set the oven to 350°F.

2. Combine the apples, almond flour, cinnamon, coconut oil, maple syrup, and salt in a medium bowl.

3. Put the mixture on a baking sheet that has been buttered.

4. 25 minutes in the oven, or until golden brown.

5. Enjoy warm servings!

Prep Time: Five minutes

Total Time: Twenty five minutes

2. Almond-banana Muffins:

Ingredients: Two mashed, ripe bananas, half a cup of almond flour, one-fourth cup of coconut flour, two tablespoons coconut oil, two tablespoons of maple syrup, half teaspoon baking soda, one-fourth teaspoon of salt.

Instructions:

1. Set the oven to 350°F.

2. Combine the mashed bananas with the maple syrup, almond flour, coconut flour, coconut oil, baking soda, and salt in a medium bowl.

3. Use coconut oil to grease a muffin pan.

4. In the muffin tin, divide the batter.

5. Bake for twenty minutes, or until golden brown.

6. Enjoy warm servings!

 Prep Time: Five minutes

Cooking Time: Twenty minutes

3. Cookies with oats and raisins:

Ingredients: A single cup of rolled oats, half-cup of almond flour, coconut oil two tablespoons, two tablespoons maple syrup, half-cup of raisins, half teaspoon baking soda, one-fourth teaspoon of salt.

Instructions:

1. Set the oven to 350°F.

2. Oats, almond flour, coconut oil, maple syrup, raisins, baking soda, and salt should all be combined in a medium basin.

3. Put coconut oil on a baking sheet and grease it.

4. Place the dough rounds on the baking sheet after cutting them out in small circles.

5. Until golden brown, bake for fifteen minutes.

6. Enjoy while warm.

Prep Time: Five minutes

Cooking Time: Fifteen minutes

4. Chocolate cake without flour:

Ingredients: Two cups chopped dark chocolate, half a cup of almond butter, two tablespoons coconut oil, two tablespoons of maple syrup, half-teaspoon of baking soda, one-fourth teaspoon of salt.

Instructions:

1. Set the oven to 350°F.

2. Chocolate should be melted over a double boiler.

3. Melted chocolate, almond butter, coconut oil, maple syrup, baking soda, and salt should all be combined in a medium basin.

4. Use coconut oil to grease an eight-inch cake pan.

5. Fill the cake pan with the batter.

6. A toothpick inserted should come out clean after twenty five minutes of baking.

7. Enjoy warm servings!

Prep Time: Ten minutes

Cooking Time: Twenty five minutes

5. Macarons with coconut:

Ingredients: Two cups of coconut shreds, two tablespoons of almond flour, two teaspoons of coconut oil, two teaspoons maple syrup, one-fourth teaspoon of salt.

Instructions:

1. Set the oven to 350°F.

2. Mix the shredded coconut, almond flour, coconut oil, maple syrup, and salt in a medium bowl.

3. Put coconut oil on a baking sheet and grease it.

4. Place the dough rounds on the baking sheet after cutting them out in small circles.

5. Bake for fifteen minutes, or until golden brown.

6. Enjoy while warm.

Prep Time: Five minutes

Cooking Time: Fifteen minutes

6. Coconut balls without baking:

Ingredients: Two cups of coconut shreds, two tablespoons of almond butter, two tablespoons coconut oil. two teaspoons maple syrup, one-fourth teaspoon of salt.

Instructions:

1. In a medium bowl, mix together the shredded coconut, almond butter, coconut oil, maple syrup and salt.

2. Shape the mixture into small balls.

3. Serve and enjoy!

Prep Time: Ten minutes

7. Chocolate Coconut Truffles:

Ingredients: One cup of dark chocolate, chopped, half cup of shredded coconut, two tablespoons coconut oil, two teaspoons maple syrup, one-fourth teaspoon of salt.

Instructions:

1. Chocolate should be melted over a double boiler.

2. In a medium bowl, mix together the melted chocolate, shredded coconut, coconut oil, maple syrup and salt.

3. Shape the mixture into small balls.

4. Refrigerate for fifteen minutes.

5. Serve and enjoy!

Prep Time: Ten minutes

Time to chill: Fifteen minutes

8. Fudge with coconut and almond butter:

Ingredients: One cup almond butter, half cup of coconut shreds, two table spoons coconut oil, two teaspoons maple syrup, one-fourth teaspoon of salt.

Instructions:

1. Use coconut oil to grease an eight-inch square pan.

2. Melt the almond butter, shredded coconut, coconut oil, maple syrup, and salt in a medium pot.

3. Spread the mixture evenly after pouring it into the pan.

4. For one hour, refrigerate.

5. Serve after being cut into little squares.

Prep Time: Ten minutes

Time to Relax: One Hour

9. Date-Coconut Squares:

Ingredients: One cup almond flour, half cup of coconut shreds, half cup soaked and chopped dates, two tablespoons coconut oil, two teaspoons maple syrup, one-fourth teaspoon of salt.

Instructions:

1. Set the oven to 350°F.

2. Use coconut oil to grease an eight-inch square pan.

3. Combine the almond flour, coconut oil, maple syrup, chopped dates, and salt in a medium bowl.

4. To fill the pan, spread the mixture.

5. Twenty five minutes in the oven, or until golden brown.

6. Serve after cutting into little squares.

Prep Time: Ten minutes

Cook Time: Twenty five minutes

10. No-Bake Chocolate Peanut Butter Bars:

Ingredients: One cup chopped dark chocolate, half-cup of peanut butter, two tablespoons coconut oil, two teaspoons maple syrup, one-fourth teaspoon of salt.

Instructions:

1. Use coconut oil to grease an eight-inch square pan.

2. Chocolate should be melted over a double boiler.

3. Melted chocolate, peanut butter, coconut oil, maple syrup, and salt should be combined in a medium basin.

4. Fill the pan with the mixture and spread uniformly.

5. For one hour, refrigerate.

6. Serve after cutting into little squares.

Prep Time: Ten minutes

Time to Relax: One Hour

SMOOTHIES

1. Green Goddess Smoothie:

Ingredients: One banana, one-fourth cup spinach, half cup pineapple, half cup coconut milk, one-fourth cup Greek yogurt , one teaspoon honey, half teaspoon ground flaxseed.

Instructions:

1. All the ingredients should be combined in a blender and blended until fully smooth.

2. Serve right away.

Prep Time: Five minutes

2. Coconut Almond Smoothie:

Ingredients: one banana, half a cup of almond milk, one-fourth cup of coconut flakes, One-fourth cup Greek yogurt, half a cup ice, one teaspoon each of honey and chia seeds.

Instructions:

1. Grind all the ingredients together in a blender until perfectly creamy.

2. Serve right away.

Prep Time: Five minutes

3. Tropical Carrot Smoothie:

Ingredients: One banana, half a cup of carrot juice, one-fourth cup spinach, half cup pineapple, one-fourth cup Greek yogurt, half teaspoon ground flaxseed and one teaspoon honey.

Instructions:

1. All the ingredients should be mixed in a blender and blended until fully smooth.

2. Serve right away.

Prep Time: Five minutes

4. Vanilla Berry Smoothie:

Ingredients: One banana, half a cup of almond milk, half a cup of frozen berries, one-fourth cup Greek yogurt, half teaspoon ground flaxseed, one teaspoon honey and one teaspoon vanilla extract.

Instructions:

1 Blend all the ingredients together in a blender, then process until totally smooth.

2. Serve right away.

Prep Time: Five minutes

5. Banana Kale Smoothie:

Ingredients: Half a cup of almond milk, one-fourth cup each of spinach and kale, one-fourth cup Greek yogurt, half teaspoon ground flaxseed and one teaspoon honey

Instructions:

1. Combine all of the ingredients in a blender and blend until fully creamy.

2. Serve right away.

Prep Time: Five minutes

6. Peanut Butter Banana Smoothie:

Ingredients: Two tablespoons of peanut butter, half cup of almond milk, one-fourth cup Greek yogurt, half teaspoon ground flaxseed and one teaspoon honey

Instructions:

1. Grind all the ingredients together in a mixer until perfectly creamy.

2. Serve right away.

Prep Time: Five minutes

7. Blueberry Banana Smoothie:

Ingredients: One banana, half a cup of almond milk, half cup blueberries frozen, one-fourth cup Greek yogurt, one spoonful of honey, half teaspoon flaxseed, ground

Instructions:

1. In a blender, add all of the ingredients and process until totally smooth.

2. Serve right away.

Prep Time: Five minutes

8. Peach Mango Smoothie:

Ingredients: One banana, half a cup of almond milk, half cup peaches frozen, half cup mangoes frozen, one-fourth cup Greek yogurt, half teaspoon ground flaxseed and one teaspoon honey.

Instructions:

1. Combine all of the ingredients in a blender and pulse until entirely creamy.

2. Serve right away.

Prep Time: Five minutes

9. An apple cinnamon smoothie:

Ingredients: One banana, half a cup of almond milk, half cup applesauce, one-fourth cup Greek yogurt, half teaspoon ground flaxseed, one teaspoon honey, and half teaspoon cinnamon.

Instructions:

1. Merge all of the items in a blender and process until totally creamy.

2. Serve right away.

Prep Time: Five minutes

10. Avocado Kale Smoothie:

Ingredients: One banana, half a cup of almond milk, one-fourth cup each of spinach and kale, one-fourth cup of Greek yogurt, half an avocado, half teaspoon ground flaxseed and one teaspoon honey.

Instructions:

1. Add all of the ingredients and grind until perfectly creamy.

2. Serve right away.

Prep Time: Five minutes

CONCLUSION

A. Key point summary: PCOS is a complicated hormonal condition that affects a large number of women of reproductive age. It can produce a number of symptoms, including irregular menstruation cycles, elevated testosterone levels, and the appearance of cysts on the ovaries. Inositol, N-Acetyl Cysteine (NAC), Vitamin D, Omega-3 Fatty Acids, Chromium, and Vitex (Chasteberry) supplements may be beneficial in treating PCOS symptoms, but it is critical to check with a healthcare expert before beginning any supplement regimen.

B. The significance of seeking medical advice: Before beginning any supplement program, contact with a healthcare expert. They can advise you on the proper dosage and ensure that the supplement is safe and appropriate for you.

C. Resources for additional information: There are numerous resources available for additional information about PCOS and PCOS supplements. Websites of recognized organizations, such as the American College of Obstetricians and Gynecologists (ACOG) and the Polycystic Ovary Syndrome Association (PCOSA), as well as publications and essays on the issue, are among them.

It's crucial to note that while supplements can help with PCOS symptoms, they are not a replacement for medical treatment. It is feasible to control PCOS and enhance overall health with the assistance of a healthcare practitioner. To ensure that the chosen treatment plan is effective, it is critical to maintain monitoring symptoms and talking with a healthcare practitioner.

www.ingramcontent.com/pod-product-compliance
Lightning Source LLC
Chambersburg PA
CBHW071139220526
45467CB00015B/1537